HOW I GOT RID OF BAD BREATH

Chemutai B. Terer

This page was intentionally left blank.

Disclaimer

This book expresses the personal opinion of the author
and may by no means be used as an alternative or
substitution to professional medical advice. The readers
are advised to use the contents of this book for
informational purposes only and seek medical attention
in advance.

Table of Contents

Dedication

This book is dedicated to all those people out there struggling with bad breath. There is a way out.

Introduction

It is very frustrating to have a condition such as bad breath and try all the possible solutions that there is but with no cure! This book contains my personal experience with bad breath and how I managed to finally get rid of it. Am going to indulge you with my experience, other ailments that I believe were associated with bad breath, the methods I tried that didn't clear the issue and finally how I got rid of Bad breath.

CHAPTER 1

My experience with Bad breath

I had a normal childhood when growing up but with frequent issues with my ear, nose and throat. This meant that I was always on antibiotics which I later discovered is not very good for the body.
I first noticed my bad breath when I was a teenager and this continued all the way into my late twenties. As it is, it affected my social interaction. If you have this condition you would know what I am talking about. Fortunately, this meant indulging in my studies which I successfully passed.
I actually stumbled upon its cure after giving birth to my firstborn son. I am hoping that too will work for you.

CHAPTER 2

Ailments that I believe were related to bad breath

In my experience with bad breath, there are a number of issues that I totally believe that were connected to my bad breath. Am going to highlight them below and these might sound familiar to what you are going through right now.

Yeast infections

If you are a lady, you would probably know more about this. It's a vaginal infection that is very irritating and you would not want to have an encounter with it! During this time, I had numerous recurrent yeast infection such that I forgot what if meant to be normal again.
I would be put on some drugs but after a small while, the infection would recur again. It was frustrating.

Constipation

Am not sure if everyone with bad breath has
this symptom. I realized that my visits to
the washroom were an uphill task. It would
leave me sometimes with tears. I would use
roughages but somehow this went on for
quite some time.

Moodiness/ irritability

My moods were all over the place. I was
easily irritated. Funny thing is that I
thought this was normal and I was just
created that way. I currently know it
different since I got rid of my bad breath

Skin rashes

I used to have some skin rashes especially on
my upper back. Well, I never gave them
much thought since, thank God! It wasn't
out there. I noticed that all the skin got
cleared once my breath got clear too.

Irregular periods

My periods would be unpredictable, one time
I would have like two periods in a month
and the other time I would be missing my
periods. Currently my periods have
stabilized and the cycle is very regular. If
you are lady and you are going through this,
there is hope. Keep reading.

CHAPTER 3

Remedies that I tried but only worked for some time

Frequent brushing of teeth after meals

It's very ironic that when you have an issue of bad breath, the more you brush your teeth the more of the stench it oozes. It is such an embarrassing thing. If you have the issue of bad breath, you understand what am talking about.
Everybody thinks that you are not doing a good job of cleaning your mouth. What they don't understand is that, your case is different. And as much its bothering them, to you is such a burden.

Use of mouth wash

The mouth wash was nice but it only worked in masking the smell for a short while. This meant that you had to keep tabs on whether the grace period has elapsed for you to go back to your usual self.

Dose of antibiotics and antifungal

I used to visit the doctors and am prescribed the antibiotics or antifungal for bad breath. These worked only for a while, when taking the medicines, but immediately am done with them, my bad breath would come back. I used to get frustrated. I would ask why don't I just brush my teeth like the others and be good to go! So yes, this too could not cure my bad breath.

Professional dental cleaning

I must admit that I was not even aware that this was a thing. I only did this when I was in my twenties and had insurance to cover the cost. Cleaning worked to remove tar and plagues but did not get rid of my bad breath. Don't get me wrong, dental cleaning helped in plague and tar removal and I would recommend it for anybody with these issues but it won't get rid of bad breath.

CHAPTER 4

What got rid of my bad breath

I came to the realization that my breath was clear after like three to five months of following this advice that am about to give you. When doing all these, my intentions were to actually lose weight for the most part of the stuff. This was after I had had a baby and gained a bunch of weight and I was not happy with the weight that I weighed back then.

Quitting processed sugar

My pregnancy came with the hatred of Sugar and anything with sugar. This helped a lot with quitting the sugar all together. I didn't know that by then that this would bring about a big change to my body and breath.
I started realizing that whenever I took processed sugar, I had some fermented taste in my mouth but immediately I stopped, the fermented taste would disappear.

I decided to totally quit sugar from then even after I gave birth to my son. I currently don't take processed sugar in my tea or any sugary beverage unless it's in its natural form example in fruit juice.

Elimination/minimizing wheat products

It is now popular knowledge that wheat products and especially the processed one is not good for the body. You can check all over the internet and you will get to know the negative effects of taking wheat products. In my quest to lose weight, I decided to remove wheat products from my diet. The results were clear breath, clear skin and reduced weight. Who wouldn't want that!

Increased water intake

I cannot stress enough on the importance of hydration in making your breath clear. When I gave birth to my son, one thing that naturally came with the breastfeeding was that I tended to need more water than normal even during the night. I would find myself taking up to four to five liters of water in a day. At first, I didn't know that this was serving to help my breath stay clear. Although now I am not breastfeeding, I continue to take two and above liters of water in a day just to keep bad breath away.

Intermittent fasting

As we all know that staying away from especially wheat products is such a tall order for many of us. Once in a while you get yourself indulging and the only way to reset or restore your balance is to do intermittent fasting while avoiding wheat. This ensures that if you lose your way, you can reset and continue with your routine.
Intermittent fasting helps your body in getting rid of toxins including bad breath. Remember to take a lot of water during your fasting to avoid dehydration.

CHAPTER 5

Wrap up

By following the advice, I have given you, I was able to get rid of my bad breath which consequently dealt with recurrent yeast infections, constipation, skin rashes and now my moods are stable and my periods are regular.

Getting rid of bad breath calls for lifestyle changes. As stated in the previous chapter, you will need to sacrifice some things. At start it will seem to be very hard for you but you need to put your focus on the benefits that you will reap in the end.

Remember to continue with taking care of your mouth hygiene and Incorporate more vegetables in your diet.

This page was intentionally left blank

Notes

Notes

Notes

www.ingramcontent.com/pod-product-compliance
Lightning Source LLC
Chambersburg PA
CBHW051143250726
48655CB00007B/3211